THE
HOMOEOPATHY
AND
BIOGRAPHICAL
SKETCH OF
HAHNEMANN

B. JAIN PUBLISHERS (P) LTD.
New Delhi-110055

THE SPIRIT OF
HOMOEOPATHY

AND

BIOGRAPHICAL SKETCH OF HAHNEMANN

Reprint Edition : 2002

Price : Rs. 30-00

Published by

Kuldeep Jain

for

B. Jain Publishers (P) Ltd.

1921, Chuna Mandi, Street No. 10,
Paharganj, New Delhi 110 055 (INDIA)
Ph: 3670430; 3670572; 3683200; 3683300
Fax: 011-3610471 & 3683400
Website: www.bjainindia.com, Email: bjain@vsnl.com

Printed in India by :
Unisons Techno Financial Consultants (P) Ltd.
522, FIE, Patpar Ganj, Delhi - 110 092

ISBN 81-7021-1122-4

BOOK CODE : BH-5568

The Spirit
of
Homoeopathy*

It is impossible to divine the internal essential nature of diseases and the changes they effect in the hidden parts of the body, and it is absurd to frame a system of treatment on such hypothetical surmises and assumptions; it is impossible to divine the medicinal properties of remedies from any chemical hypotheses or from their smell, colour or taste, and it is absurd to attempt, from such hypothetical surmises and assumptions, to apply to the treatment of diseases these substances, which are so hurtful when wrongly administered. And even were such practice ever so customary and ever so generally in use, were it even the *only one in vogue* for thousands of years, it would nevertheless

---

* [This essay, written by Hahnemann as long ago as 1813, nearly three years after the publication of the *Organon*, and intended by him as a popular exposition of his system, is well worth perusal at the present day; as in essentials the homoeopathic system still remains as it was after it had been finally determined on by its author after seventeen years of arduous study and experiment. In practice, of course, homoeopathy has gained vastly since that time by the great increase of the materia medica, containing the instruments it employs, through the labours of Hahnemann and his disciples.]

continue to be a senseless and pernicious practice to found on empty surmises our idea of the morbid condition of the interior, and to attempt to combat this with equally imaginary properties of medicines.

Appreciable, distinctly appreciable to our senses must that be which is to be removed in each disease in order to transform it into health, and right clearly must each remedy express what it can positively cure, if medical art is to cease to be a wanton game of hazard with human life, and to commence to be the sure deliverer from diseases.

I will now show what there is undeniably curable in disease, and how the curative properties of medicines are to be distinctly perceived and employed for curative purposes.

●   ●   ●

What life is can only be known empirically from its phenomena and manifestations, but no conception of it can be formed by any metaphysical speculations *a priory*; what life is, in its actual essential nature, can never be perceived by mortal man, nor ascertained by speculative ratiocination.

To the explanation of human life, as also its twofold conditions, health and disease, the principles by which we explain other phenomena are quite inapplicable. With nought in the world can we compare it save with itself alone; neither with a piece of clockwork, nor with a hydraulic machine, nor with chemical processes, nor with decompositions and recompositions of gases, nor with a galvanic battery; in short, with nothing destitute of life. Human life is *in no respect* regulated by purely physical laws, which only obtain among inorganic substances. The material substances of which the human organism is composed no longer follow, in this vital combination, the laws to which material substances in the inanimate condition are subject; they are regulated by the laws peculiar to vitality alone; they are themselves animated and vitalised just as the whole system is animated and vitalised. Here a nameless fundamental power reigns omnipotent, which abrogates all the tendency of the component parts of the body to obey the laws of gravitation, of momentum, of the *vis inertiae*, of fermentation, of putrefaction, etc., and brings them under subjection to the wonderful laws of life alone-in other words, maintains them in the condition of *sensibility* and *activity* necessary to the preservation of the living whole, a condition almost spiritually dynamic.

Now, as the condition of the organism and its health depend solely on the health of the life which animates it, in like manner it follows that the altered health, which we term disease, consists of a condition altered originally only in its vital sensibilities and functions, irrespective of all chemical or mechanical considerations; that is to say, it must consist in a dynamically altered condition, a changed mode of being, whereby a change in the properties of the material component parts of the body is afterwards effected, which is a necessary consequence of the morbidly altered condition of the living whole in every individual case.

Moreover, the influence of morbific noxae, which for the most part excite from without the various maladies in us, is generally so invisible and so immaterial,[1] that it is impossible that it can *immediately* either mechanically disturb or derange the component parts of our body in their form and substance, or infuse any pernicious acrid fluid into our blood vessels whereby the mass of our humours can be chemically altered and depraved—an inadmissible quite improbable, crass conception of mechanical minds. The exciting causes of disease rather act by means of their virtual- quality on the state of our life (on our health) only in a dynamic, almost spiritual, manner; and inasmuch as they first derange the organs of the higher rank and of the vital force, there occurs from this state of derangement, from this dynamic alteration of the living whole, an altered sensation (uneasiness, pains) and an altered activity (abnormal functions) of each individual organ and of all of them collectively, whereby there must also be necessity secondarily occur alteration of the juices in our vessels and secretion of abnormal matters, the inevitable consequence of the altered vital character, which now differs from the healthy state.

These abnormal matters that show themselves in diseases are consequently merely products of the disease itself, which, as long as the malady retains its present character, must of necessity be secreted, and thus constitute a portion of the morbid phenomena (symptoms);

1 With the exception of a few surgical affections and the disagreeable effects produced by indigestible foreign substances, which sometimes find their way into the intestinal canal.

they are merely effects, and therefore manifestations, of the existing internal ill-health, and they do certainly not react (although they often contain the infecting principle for other, healthy individuals) upon the diseased body that produced them, as disease-exciting or maintaining substances, that is, as material morbific causes,[1] just as a person cannot infect other parts of his own body at the same time with the virus from his own chancre or with the gonorrhoeal matter from his own urethra, or increase his disease therewith, or as a viper cannot inflict on itself a fatal or a dangerous bite with its own poison.

Hence, it is obvious that the diseases of human beings excited by the dynamic and virtual influence of morbific noxae can be originally only dynamical derangements (caused almost solely by a spiritual process) of the vital character of our organism.

We readily perceive that these dynamic derangements of the vital character of our organism which we term diseases, since they are nothing else than altered sensations and functions, can also express themselves by nothing but by an aggregate of symptoms, and only as such are they cognizable to our powers of observation.

Now, as in a profession of such importance to

---

1 Hence by scouring out and mechanically removing these abnormal matters, acridities and morbid organisations, their source, the disease itself, can just as little be cured as a coryza can be shortened or cured by blowing the nose as frequently and as thoroughly as possible; it lasts not a day longer than its proper course, although the nose should not be cleansed by blowing it at all.

human life as medicine is, nothing but the state of the diseased body plainly cognizable by our perceptive faculties can be recognised as the object of cure, and ought to guide our steps (to prefer to be guided here by conjectures and undemonstrable hypotheses would be dangerous folly, nay crime and treason against humanity), it follows, that since diseases, as dynamic derangements of the vital character, express themselves *solely* by alterations of the sensations and functions of our organism, that is, *solely* by an aggregate of perceptible symptoms, this alone can be the object of treatment in every case of disease. *For when all morbid symptoms are removed, nothing remains but health.*

Now, because diseases are only dynamic derangements of our health and vital character, they cannot be removed by man otherwise than by means of agents and powers which also are capable of producing dynamical derangements of the human health, that is to say, diseases are cured virtually and dynamically by medicines.[1]

---

1 Not by means of pretended solvent or mechanically dispersing, clearing-out and expulsive powers of medicinal substances; not by means of a (blood-purifying, humour-improving) power they possess of electively expelling imaginary morbific principles; not by means of any antiseptic power they have (such as is efficacious in dead, putrefying flesh); not by chemical or physical action of any other imaginable sort, such as takes place in dead material things, as has hither to been falsely imagined and dreamt by the various medical schools.

The more modern schools have indeed began in some

These active substances and powers (medicines which we have at our service, effect the cure of diseases by means of the same dynamic power of altering the actual state of health, by means of the same power of deranging the vital character of our organism in respect of its sensations and functions, by which they are able to affect also the healthy individual, to produce in him dynamic changes and certain morbid symptoms, the knowledge of which, as we shall see, affords us the most trustworthy information concerning the morbid states that can be most certainly cured by each particular medicine. Hence, nothing in the world can accomplish a cure, no substance, no power can effect a change in the human organism of such a character as that the disease shall yield to it, except a force capable

---

degree to regard disease as dynamic derangements, and their intention, too, is to remove them in some sort of dynamical way by medicines, but inasmuch as they fail to perceive that the sensible, irritable and reproductive activity of life is *in mode of qualitate* susceptible of an infinity of changes, and as they do not regard the innumerable varieties of morbid signs (that infinity of internal alterations only congnizable by us in their reflex) for what they actually are, to wit, the only reliable object for treatment; but as they only hypothetically recognise an abnormal increase and decrease of their dimensions *quoad quantitatem,* and *in an equally arbitrary manner* confide to the medicines they employ the task of changing to the normal state this one-sided increase and decrease, and thereby curing them; they thus have in their mind nothing but false ideas, both of the object of cure and of the properties of the medicines.

of absolutely (dynamically) deranging the human health, consequently also of morbidly altering its healthy state.[1]

On the other hand, however, there is also no agent, no power in nature capable of morbidly affecting the healthy individual, which does not at the same time possess the faculty of curing certain morbid states.

Now, as the power of curing diseases, as also of morbidly affecting the healthy, is met with in inseparable combination in all medicines, and as both these properties evidently spring from one and the same source, namely, from their power of dynamically deranging human health, and as it is hence impossible that they can act according to a different inherent natural law in the sick to that according to which they act on the health; it follows that it must be the same power of the medicine that cures the disease in the sick as produces the morbid symptoms in the healthy.[2]

Hence, also we shall find that the curative power of medicines, and what each of them is able to effect in diseases, expresses itself in no other mode in the world so surely and palpably, and cannot be ascertained by us in any purer and more perfect manner than by the morbid phenomena and symptoms (the kinds of artificial diseases) which the medicines develop in healthy individuals. For once we have before us records of the peculiar (artificial) morbid symptoms produced by the

---

1 Consequently no substance, for example, that is purely nutritious.

2 The different results in these two cases is owing solely to the difference of the object that has to be altered.

various medicines on healthy individuals, we only require a series of pure trials to decide what medicinal symptoms will always rapidly and permanently cure and remove certain symptoms of disease, in order to know, in every case before hand, which of all the different medicines, known and thoroughly tested as to their peculiar symptoms, must be the most certain remedy in every case of disease.[1]

---

1 Simple, true, and natural as this maxim is, so much so that one would have imagined it would long since have been adopted as the rule for ascertaining the curative powers of drugs, it is yet a fact that nothing the least like it has hitherto been thought of. During the several thousands of years over which history extends, no one hit upon this natural method of first ascertaining the curative powers of medicines before giving them in diseases. In all ages down to the present times it was imagined that the curative powers of medicines could be learned in no other way than from the result of their employment in disease themselves (*ab usu in morbis*); it was sought to learn them from those cases where a certain medicine (more frequently a combination of various medicines) had been found serviceable in a particular case of disease. But even from the efficacious result of one single medicine given in a case of disease accurately described (which but rarely happened), we never can know the case in which that medicine would again prove serviceable, because (with the exception of diseases caused by miasms of a fixed character, as smallpox, measles, syphilis, itch, etc. and those arising from various noxae that always remain the same, as *rheumatic gout*, etc.), all other cases of disease are mere individualities, that is to say, all present themselves in nature with different combinations of symptoms, have never before occurred, and can never again occur in exactly the same manner;

If, then, we ask experience what artificial diseases
(observed to be produced by medicines) can be
beneficially employed against certain natural morbid

consequently, because a medicine has cured one case
we cannot thence infer that it will cure another (different)
case. The forced arrangement of these cases of disease
(which nature in her wisdom produces in endless variety)
under certain nosological heads, as is arbitrarily done
by pathology, is an unreal human performance, which
leads to constant fallacies and to the confounding together
of very different states.

Equally misleading and entrust worthy, although in
all ages universally practised, is the determination of
the general (curative) action of medicines from certain
effects following their employment in diseases; when,
for example, in some cases of disease *during* the use of
a medicine, (generally mixed up with others) there
sometimes occurred a more copious secretion of urine
or perspiration, the catamenia came on, convulsions
ceased, there occurred a kind of sleep, expectoration,
etc., the medicine (to which the honour was attributed
more than to the others in the mixture) was instantly
elevated by the materia medica to the rank of a diuretic,
a diaphoretic, an emmenagogue, an antispasmodic, a
soporific, an expectorant, and thereby not only was a
fallacium causo committed by confounding the word *during*
with *by*, but quite a false conclusion was drawn, a
particulari ad universale, in opposition to all the laws of
reason; indeed the conditional was made unconditional.
For a substance that does not in every case of disease
promote urine and perspiration, that does not in every
instance bring on the catamenia and sleep, that does
not subdue all convulsions, and cause every cough to
come to expectoration, cannot be said by a person of
sound reason to be nonconditionally and absolutely

states; if we ask it whether the change to health (cure) may be expected to ensure most certainly and in the most permanent manner :–

(1)   By the use of such medicines as are capable of producing in the healthy body a *different* (alloeopathic) affection from that exhibited by the disease to be cured;

(2)   Or by the employment of such as are capable of exciting in the healthy individual an *opposite* (enantiopathic, antipathic) state to that of the case to be cured;

(3)   Or by the administration of such medicines as can cause a *similar* (homoeopathic) state to the natural disease before us (for these are the only three possible modes of employing them), experience speaks indubitably for the last method.

But it is moreover self-evident that medicines which act *heterogeneously* and *alloeopathically*, which tend to develop in the healthy subject different symptoms from those presented by the disease to be cured, from the very nature of things can never be suitable and

---

diuretic, diaphoretic, emmenagogue, soporific, antispas-modic and expectorant! And yet this is, what the ordinary materia medica does. Indeed it is impossible that in the complex phenomena of our health, in the multifarious combinations of different symptoms presented by the innumerable varieties of human diseases, the employ-ment of a remedy can exhibit its pure, original medicinal effect, and exactly what we can expect it to do for derange-ments of our health. These can only be shown by medicines given to persons in health.

efficacious in this case, but they must act awry,
otherwise all diseases must necessarily be cured in a
rapid, certain and permanent manner by all medicines,
however they may differ. Now as every medicine
possesses an action different from that of every other,
and as, according to eternal natural laws, every disease
causes a derangement of the human health different
from that caused by all other diseases this proposition
contains an innate contradiction (*contradictionem in
adjecto*), and is self-demonstrative of the impossibility
of a good result, since every given change can only be
effected by an adequate cause, but not per *quamlibet
causam*. And daily experience also proves that the
ordinary practice of prescribing complex recipes
containing a variety of unknown medicines in diseases,
does indeed do many things, but very rarely cures.

The second mode of treating diseases by medicines
is the employment of an agent capable of altering the
existing derangement of the health (the disease, or most
prominent morbid symptom) in an *enantiopathic,
antipathic*, or *contrary* manner (the *palliative* employment
of a medicine). Such an employment, as will be readily
seen, cannot effect a permanent cure of the disease,
because the malady must soon afterwards recur, and
that in an aggravated degree. The process that takes
place is as follows :–

According to a wonderful provision of nature,
organised living beings are not regulated by the laws of
unorganised (dead) physical matter, they do not receive
the influence of external agents, like the latter, in a
passive manner, they do not like the latter, yield

themselves docilely to external impressions, but strive
to set up the opposite of this effect.[1] The living human
body does indeed allow itself to be in the first instance
changed by the action of physical forces; but this change
is not in it, as in inorganic substances permanent (–as
it ought necessarily to be if the medicinal force acting
in a *contrary manner* to the disease could produce a

---

1 The expressed, green juice of plants, which is in that
   state no longer living, when spread upon linen cloth is
   soon bleached and its colour annihilated by exposure to
   sunlight, whereas the colourless living plant that has
   been kept in a dark cellar, soon recovers its full green
   colour when exposed to the same sunlight. A root dug
   up and dried (dead), if buried in a warm and damp soil,
   rapidly undergoes complete decomposition and
   destruction, whilst a living root in the same warm damp
   soil sends forth gay sprouts.—Foaming malt beer in full
   fermentation rapidly turns to vinegar when exposed to
   a temperature of 96° Fahr. in a jar, but in the healthy
   human stomach at the same temperature the
   fermentation ceases, and it soon becomes converted into
   a mild nutritious juice.—Half-decomposed and strong-
   smelling game as also beef and other flesh meat, partaken
   of by a healthy individual, furnish excrement with the
   least amount of odour, whereas cinchona bark, which is
   calculated powerfully to check decomposition in lifeless
   animal substances, is acted against by the intestines in
   such a manner that the most foetid flatus is developed.—
   Mild carbonate of lime removes all acidity from inorganic
   matter, but when taken into the healthy stomach sour
   perspiration usually ensues.—Whilst the dead animal
   fibre is preserved by nothing more certainly and powerfully than by tannin, clean ulcers in a living individual,
   when they are frequently dressed with tannin, become

permanent effect, a *durable* benefit–); on the contrary, the living human organism strives to develop by antagonism the exact opposite of the affection first produced in it from without[1]—as for instance, a hand kept long enough in ice-cold water, after being withdrawn does not remain cold, nor merely assume the temperature of the surrounding atmosphere, as a stone (dead) ball would do, or even resume the temperature of the rest of the body, no ! the colder the water of the bath was, and the longer it acted on the healthy skin of the hand, the more *inflamed* and hotter does the latter afterwards become.

Therefore, it cannot but happen that a medicine having an action opposite to the symptoms of the disease, will reverse the morbid symptoms for but a very short time, but must soon yield to the antagonism inherent in the living body, which produces an opposite state, that is to say, a state the direct contrary of that transient delusive state of the health effected by the palliative, and one corresponding to the original malady, which constitutes an actual addition to the now recurring, uneradicated, original affection, and is

unclean, green and putrid. A hand plunged into warm water becomes subsequently colder than the hand that has not been so treated and it becomes colder the warmer the water was.

1 This is the law of nature in obedience to which, the employment of every medicine produces at first certain dynamic changes and morbid symptoms in the living human body (*primary* or *first action of the medicines*), but on the other hand, by means of a peculiar antagonism (which may in many instances be termed the effort of

consequently an increased degree of the original disease. And thus the malady is always *certainly* aggravated, after the palliative—the medicine that acts in an opposite and enantiopathic manner—has exhausted its action.

In chronic diseases—the injurious character of the antagonistically-acting (palliative) remedy often displays itself in a high degree, since from its repeated exhibition, in order that it should merely produce its delusive effect (a very transient semblance of health), it must be administered in larger doses, which are often productive of serious danger to life, or even of actual death.

There remains, therefore, only a *third* mode of employing medicines in order to effect a really beneficial result, to wit, by employing in every case such an one as tends to excite of itself an artificial, morbid affection in the organism *similar* (homoeopathic), best if very *similar,* to the actual case of disease.

That this mode of employing medicines is, and must of necessity be, the only best method, can easily be proved by reasoning, as it has also already been confirmed both by innumerable experiences of physicians who practise according to my doctrines, and by daily experience.

It will, therefore, not be difficult to perceive what are the laws of nature according to which the only appropriate cure of diseases, the homoeopathic, takes place, and must necessarily take place.

---

self-preservation), produces a state the very opposite of the first (the *secondary* or *after action*), as for instance, in the case of narcotic substances, insensibility is produced in the primary action, sensitiveness to pain in the secondary.

The first of these unmistakable laws of nature is *the susceptibility of the living organism for natural diseases is incomparably less than it is for medicinal diseases.*

A multitude of disease-exciting causes act daily and hourly upon us, but they are incapable of deranging the equilibrium of the health, or of making the healthy sick; the activity of the life-sustaining power within us usually withstands the most of them, the individual remains healthy. It is only when these external noxae assail us in a very aggravated degree, and we are especially exposed to their influence, that we get ill, but even then we only become seriously ill when our organism has a particularly impressionable, weak side (predisposition), that makes it more disposed to be affected and its health deranged by the existing (simple or compound) morbific cause.

If the inimical physical and psychical forces in nature, which are termed morbific noxae, possessed an unconditional power of deranging the human health, they would, as they are universally distributed, not leave any one in good health; everyone would be ill, and we should never be able to obtain an idea of health. But as, taken on the whole diseases are only exceptional states of the human health, and it is necessary that such a number of circumstances and conditions, as regards both the morbific forces and the individual to be affected with disease, should conjoin before a disease is produced by its exciting causes, it follows, *that the individual is so little liable to be affected by such noxae, that they can never unconditionally make him ill, and*

*that the human organism is capable of being deranged
to disease by them only in consequence of a particular
predisposition.*

But it is far otherwise with the artificial dynamic
forces which we term medicines. For every true medicine
acts at *all* times, under *all* circumstances, on *every*
living, animated body, and excites in it the symptoms
peculiar to it (even in a way perceptible to the senses
if the dose be large enough) so that *evidently every living
human organism must always and inevitably be affected
by the medicinal disease and, as it were, infected,* which,
as is well known, is not the case with respect to natural
diseases.

All experience proves, incontestably that the
human body is much more apt and disposed to be
affected by medicinal forces and to have its health
deranged by them, then by the morbific noxae and
contagious miasmas, or, what is the same thing, that
the medicinal forces possess an absolute power of
deranging human health, whereas the morbific agents
possess only a very conditional power, over which the
former can exercise a pre-ponderating influence.

To this circumstance it is owing that medicines
are able to cure diseases at all (that is to say, we see
that the morbid affection may be eradicated from the
diseased organism, if the latter be subjected to the
appropriate alteration by means of medicine); but in
order that the cure should take place, the second natural
law should also be fulfilled, to wit, *a stronger dynamic
affection permanently extinguishes the weaker in the*

living organism, provided the former be similar in kind to the latter, for the dynamic alteration of the health to be anticipated from the medicine should, as I think I have proved, neither *differ in kind* from, that is, be *alloeopathic* to the morbid derangement, in order that, as happens in the ordinary mode of practice, a still greater derangement may not ensue; nor should be *opposite* to it, in order that a merely palliative delusive amelioration may not ensure, to be followed by an inevitable aggravation of the original malady; but the medicine must have been proved by observations to possess the tendency to develop of itself a state of health *similar* to the disease (be able to excite similar symptoms in the healthy body), in order to be a remedy of permanent efficacy.

Now, as the dynamic affections of the organism (caused by disease or by medicine) are only cognizable by the phenomena of altered function and altered sensation, and consequently the similarity of its dynamic affections to one another can only express themselves by similarity of symptoms; but as the organism (as being much more readily deranged by medicine than by disease) must yield more to the medicinal affection, that is to say, must be more disposed to allow itself to be influenced and deranged by medicine than by the similar natural morbid affection, it follows undeniably, that it will be freed from the natural morbid affection if we allow it to be acted on by a medicine which, while differing in its nature from the disease, resembles it very closely in the symptoms it causes, that is to say, is homoeopathic; for the organism, as a living, individual unity, cannot receive two similar dynamic affections at the same time, without the weaker yielding to the stronger similar one; consequently, as it is more disposed to be more strongly affected by the one (the medicinal affection), the other, similar, weaker one (the natural morbid affection) must necessarily give way; and thereby the organism is cured of its disease.

Let it not be imagined that the living organism, if a new similar affection be communicated to it when diseased by a dose of homoeopathic medicine, will be thereby more seriously deranged, that is, burdened with an addition to its sufferings, just as a leaden plate already pressed upon by an iron weight is still more severely squeezed by placing a stone in addition upon it; or as a piece of copper heated by friction must become still hotter by pouring on it water at a more elevated temperature. No, our living organism does not behave passively, it is not subject to the laws that govern dead matter; it reacts by vital antagonism, so as to surrender itself as an individual living whole to its morbid derangement, and to allow this to be extinguished within it when a stronger affection of a similar kind, produced in it by homoeopathic medicine, takes possession of it.

Such a spiritually reacting being is our living human organism, which with automatic power expels from itself a weaker derangement (disease), whenever the stronger force of the homoeopathic medicine produces in it another but very similar affection; or in other words, which, on account of the unity of its life, cannot suffer at the same time from two similar general derangements, but must discard the previous dynamic affection (disease), whenever it is acted on by a second dynamic force (medicine), more capable of deranging it, that has a great resemblance to the former in its power of affecting the state of health (its symptoms). Something similar takes place in the human mind.

But as the human organism even in health is more capable of being affected by medicine than by disease, as I have shown above, so when it is diseased, it is beyond comparison more affectable by homoeopathic medicine than by any other (whether alloeopathic or enantiopathic), and indeed it is *affectable in the highest degree*; since, as it is already disposed and excited by the disease to certain symptoms, it must now be more susceptible of the altering influence of similar symptoms (by the homoeopathic medicine)—just as similar mental affections render the mind very sensitive to similar emotions—hence only the *smallest dose* of them is *necessary* and *useful* for the cure, that is for altering the diseased organism into the similar medicinal disease; and *a greater dose is not necessary* on this account also, because the spiritual power of the medicine does not in this instance accomplish its object by means of quantity, but by potentiality and quality (dynamic fitness, homoeopathy)—and *a greater dose is not useful*, but on the contrary *injurious*, because whilst the larger dose, on the one hand, does not dynamically overpower the morbid affection more certainly than the smallest dose of the most appropriate medicine, on the other hand it imposes a complex medicinal disease in its place, which is always a malady, though it passes off after a certain time.

Hence, the organism will be powerfully affected and taken possession of by the force of even a very small dose of a medicinal substance, which, by its tendency to excite similar symptoms, can outweigh and extinguish the totality of the symptoms of the disease; it becomes, as I have said, free from the morbid affection at the very instant that it is taken possession of by the medicinal affection, by which it is much more liable to be altered.

Now, as medicinal forces do of themselves, even in larger doses, keep the healthy organism for a few days only under their influence, it will readily be conceived that a small dose, and in acute diseases a very small dose of them (as has been shown to be necessary in homoeopathic treatment), can only affect the system for a short time; the smallest doses, indeed, in acute diseases, only for a few hours; and then the medicinal affection that has taken the place of the disease passes unobservedly and very rapidly into perfect health.

In the permanent cure of diseases by medicines in living organisms, nature seems never to act otherwise than in accordance with these—her manifest laws and then indeed she acts, if we may use the expression, with mathematical certainty. *There is no case of dynamic disease in the world* (excepting the death struggle, old age, if it can be considered a disease, and the destruction of some indispensable viscus or member), *whose symptoms can be met with in great similarity among the positive effects of a medicine, which will not be rapidly and permanently cured by this medicine.* The diseased individual can be freed from his malady in no more easy, rapid, certain, reliable and permanent manner, by any conceivable mode of treatment, than by means of the homoeopathic medicine in small doses.

Biographical Sketch of Hahnemann

(Born, the 10th April, 1775. Died, the 2nd July, 1843)

—*DR. R.E. DUDGEON, M.D.*

The histories of many men who have risen to eminence in some particular branch of science teach us that they have done so under the most unfavourable circumstances and in spite of the greatest obstacles thrown in their way by fortune and by their own natural guardians. Hahnemann belonged to this class of great men.

His father, an industrious but fortuneless painter on porcelain in the celebrated manufactory at Meissen, a charming little town on the banks of the Elbe, near Dresden, discouraged all his endeavours to qualify himself for a calling superior to that he himself pursued, though he seems in other respects to have had a great influence on the character of his son by his exhortations to him exercise his independent judgement in all cases, and not to take anything on trust, but in every case to act as reflection told him was for the best. "*Prove all things, hold fast that which is good,*" was the substance of his advice. By this advice Hahnemann profited, and, notwithstanding his father's prohibition to study, he pursued his strong inclination to do so in spite of all opposition, and on many an occasion when it was thought he was sound asleep, he was consuming the midnight oil over his books, in a lamp which he had himself constructed out of clay, as he was apprehensive being discovered had he used one of the household candlesticks. This little incident I have thought worth mentioning, as it exhibits his perseverance and indomitable steadfastness of purpose even at that early age. His aptitude for study excited the admiration of his schoolmaster, with whom be became a favourite, and who undertook to direct his studies, and encouraged him to a higher order of study than that which constituted the usual curriculum of a Grammar School. This did not please his father, who several times removed him from the school and set him to some less intellectual work, but at length restored him to his favourite studies at the earnest request of his teacher, who, to meet the pecuniary difficulty, instructed the young Samuel until his twentieth year without remuneration.

On leaving school it was the custom to write an essay on some subject, and Hahnemann selected the somewhat unusual one of "*the wonderful structure of the human hand*", a theme which has in our own time been so beautifully discoursed upon by **Sir Charles Bell**, in his **Bridgewater Treatise**. Who would not like to see how the boy Hahnemann treated this subject, his selection of which shows a strong bias towards natural science?

Twenty thalers (about £ 3 sterling the only patrimony he ever received) and his father's blessing, were all he carried with him from Messen to Leipzic, where it was his intention to study medicine. He was allowed free access to the various classes, and managed to support himself by teaching French and German and by translating books from the English. From Leipzic he journeyed to Vienna, in order to witness the practice of medicine in the hospitals there, and had the good fortune to secure the friendship of **Dr. Von Quarin**, who treated him like a son, and took great pains to teach him the art of medicine. By some roguery or other, however, he lost the greater part of his money here, and so, after a sojourn in Vienna of only three quarters of a year, he found himself forced to accept the situation of family physician and librarian to the **Governor of Transylvania**, with whom he resided in Hermannstadt two years and whence he removed to graduate in Erlangen, in 1779.

"*The longing of a Swiss for his rugged Alps,*" he says, in an autobiographical fragment he has left behind him, "*cannot be more irresistible than that of a Saxon for his fatherland.*" Accordingly to fatherland he went, and settled down to practice in a small town named Hettstadt, but as there was no field for practice there, he removed, after three quarters of a year's residence, to Dessau, in 1783. Here it was, he tells us, that he first turned his attention to chemistry ; but at the end of this year he was appointed district physician in Gommern, wither he removed, and here married his first wife, whose acquaintance he had previously made

in Dessau, she being the daughter of an apothecary of
that town : here also he wrote his first book on medicine,
which gives the result of his experience of practice in
Transylvania and takes rather a desponding view of
medical practice in gernal, and of his own in particular,
as he candidly admits that most of his cases would
have done better had he let them alone. After remaining
nearly three years in Gommern—where, he naively
observes, "*no physician had ever been before, and whose
inhabitants had no desire for one*"—he transferred his
residence to Dresden; but with the exception of taking
for a year the post of physician to the hospital, during
the illness of **Dr. Wagner**, he does not seem to have
done much in the way of practice here. During the last
four years he lived in Dresden and the neighbouring
village of Lockowitz he published many chemical works,
the most celebrated of which is *a treatise upon poisoning
by arsenic*, which is quoted to this day as an authority
by the best writers on toxicology. This was probably
the period he alludes to, in his letter to Hufeland, as
that when he retired disgusted with the uncertainty of
medical practice and devoted himself to chemistry and
literature. That he made considerable progress in the
former science, his valuable tests for ascertaining the
purity of wine and of drugs and this treatise on arsenic
testify; and we have likewise the testimony of the
Swedish oracle of chemistry. Berzelius, who, knowing
well the value of Hahnemann's services to his own
science, is reported to have said, "*This man would have
been a great chemist, had he not turned a great quack.*"
We may take Berzelius's opinion as to Hahnemann's
skill in chemistry; but try his physic by other than
chemical tests.

In 1789 he removed to Leipzic, and in that year published his *treatise on Syphilis*, written the year before in Lockowitz which, I must confess, betrays no lack of confidence in the powers of medicine, and shows an intimate acquaintance with the best works of that period on the subject. But what this work is chiefly remarkable for, is its description of a new preparation, known to this day in Germany by the name of *Hahnemann's soluble mercury*, and some very novel views relative to the treatment of syphilis; the dose of mercury to be given (which is remarkably small), the signs when enough has been ingested for the cure of the diseases, and the denunciation of the local treatment of the primary sore. In 1790 he translated **Cullen's Materia Medica**, and discovered the fever-producing property of cinchona bark; which was to him what the falling apple was to Newton, and the swinging lamp in the Baptistery at Pisa, to Galileo. From this single experiment his mind appears to have been impressed by the conviction, that the pathogenetic effects of medicines would give the key to their therapeutic powers. He seems, however, to have contented himself with hunting up in the works of the ancient authors for hints respecting the physiological action of different substances, and to have tested them but sparingly, if at all, on his own person or on his friends; and in his researches, to have looked more for the peculiar and striking effects of the drugs than for those minute shades of symptoms which we find he so carefully recorded in his later years. In fact, he seems rather to have searched for parallels to those abstract forms of disease described in the works on nosology, than for analogues to the individual concrete cases of actual practice. I think any one who will read his first *Essay on a New Principle*, published in 1796, and the two papers, on *Continued and Remittant Fevers*, and on *Hebdomadal Diseases*, published in 1798, will agree with me in this opinion.

However, to return to our history Hahnemann seems to have had little or no opportunity to test his ideas by practice in Leipzic and the little village of Stotteritz close by, and must have been completely occupied with his chemical lucubrations and translation; for he wrote at his period a large number of chemical essays, and translated several chemical and other works, besides Cullen's just named. His diligence must have been something extraordinary at this time, and no doubt his increasing family was a source of great anxiety to him, and caused him to slave to the extent of which we have evidence from his publications. How sorely the 'res angusta domi' must now have pressed on Hahnemann, longing as he was for the opportunity to pursue the investigations of which he had just discovered the clue, how his great but impatient soul must have chafed and fretted at that oppressive clog of poverty— that necessity for providing bread for the daily wants of his children, which hindered him from soaring on his eagle flight into unexplored, undreamt—of regions of discovery ! And the poverty which Hahnemann endured was not merely an income so small as to prohibit an indulgence in the luxuries of life, but often, very often, and actual want of the common necessaries of existence; and this with all the anxiety of an increasing and helpless family of young children ! And yet had it not been for his poverty, Hahnemann had probably never made the discovery on which his fame built. Naturalists tell us that the oyster forms the lustrous pearl round certain extraneous substances that intrude themselves within the cavity of its shell, and irritate and vex its tender flesh—and so it is with the great and good; the vexation and annoyances of life are often the means of eliciting and developing those pearls of the mind that we admire and marvel at.

With what eagerness must not Hahnemann now have accepted the offer of the reigning Duke of Saxe Gotha to take the charge of an asylum for the insane in Georgenthal, in the Thuringian forest,—a charge which would give him a present competency, and, above all, leisure his how painfully interesting investigations, and an opportunity of putting his discovery to the test. Here, then, we find him settled for a time in 1792. A cure that he made in this institution of the Hanoverian minister Klokenburg, who had been rendered insane by a satire of Kotzebue's, created, we are told, some sensation; and, from the account he published in 1796 of this case, we find that he was one of the earliest, if not the very first advocate for that system of the insane by mildness instead of coercion which has become all but universal. "*I never allow any insane person*", he writes, "*to be punished by blows or other painful corporeal inflictions, since there can be no punishment where there is no sense of responsibility; and since such patients cannot be improved, but must be rendered worse, by such rough treatment*". May we not, then, justly claim for Hahnemann the honour of being the first who advocated and practised the moral treatment of the insane? At all events, he may divide this honour with Pineal; for we find that towards the end of this same year 1792, when Hahnemann was applying his principle of moral treatment to practice, Pineal made his first experiment of unchaining the maniacs in the Bicetre. Hahnemann does not seem to have remained long in this situation; for the same year he removed to Walshleben, where he wrote the first part of the *Friend of Health*, a popular miscellany, on hygiene principally, and the first part of his *Pharmaceutical Lexicon*, and in 1794 he went first to Pyrmont, a little watering-place in Westphalia, and thereafter to Brunswick.

In 1795 he migrated to Wolfenbuttel, and thence to Konigslutter, where he remained until 1799. In this interval of comparative settlement he gave out the second parts of his *Friend of Health* and *Pharmaceutical Lexicon*; and he had leisure to pursue his investigations and to write, in 1796, for his friend Hufeland's Journal, that remarkable *Essay on a New Principle for ascertain-ing the Remedial Powers of Medicinal Substances*, wherein he modestly but firmly expresses his belief that, for chronic diseases at least, medicines should be employed that have the power of producing similar affections in the healthy body; and the following year he published in the same journal an interesting case illustrative of his views; and wrote another essay on the irrationality of complicated systems of diet and regimen, and complex prescriptions. Several other essays followed this in rapid succession among which I may mention that on antidotes, and those on the treatment of fevers and periodical diseases. But already the hostility of his colleagues began to display itself, Hahnemann, who had now abandoned the complicated medication of absurdity of giving complex mixtures of medicines which he now invariably administered alone. The physicians of Konigslutter, jealous of the rising fame of the innovator, incited the apothecaries to bring an action against him for interfering with their privileges by dispensing his own medicines. It was in vain Hahnemann appealed to their letter and spirit of the law regulating the apothecaries' business, and argued, that their privileges only extended to the compounding of medicines, but that every man, and therefore still more every medical man, had the right to give or sell uncompounded drugs, which were the only things he employed, and which he administered, moreover, gratuitously. All in vain; the apothecaries and their allies, his jealous brethren, were too powerful for him; and contrary to law, justice, and common sense, Hahne-mann, who had shown himself a master of the apothecaries' art by his learned and laborious *Pharmaceutical Laxicon*, was prohibited from dispensing his own simple medicines.

During the last year of his residence in Konigslutter he witnessed a severe epidemic of scarlet fever, and made his glorious discovery of the prophylactic power of *Belladonna* in this disease, which alone would have sufficed to make his name remembered with gratitude by posterity. The mode of his discovery of this prophylactic is a true specimen of inductive philosophy, much more so than Jenner's somewhat similar discovery of the prophylactic power of vaccination. Knowing the power of *Belladonna* to produce a state similar to the first stage of scarlet-fever, he used it with great success at that period of the disease, and whilst his mind was occupied with the great remedial virtue he observed it to possess, a circumstance occurred which led him to believe that it was not only curative, but a preventive medicine for that malady. In a family of four children, three sickened with the disease, but the fourth, who was taking *Belladonna* at the time for an affection of the finger-joints, escaped, though she had heretofore been always the first to take any epidemic that was going about. An opportunity soon presented itself of putting its prophylactic power to the test. In a family of eight children, three were seized with the epidemic, and he immediately gave to the remaining five children *Belladonna* in small doses, and, as he had anticipated, all these five escaped the disease, not withstanding their constant exposure to the virulent emanations from their sick sisters. The epidemic presented him with numerous opportunities of verifying this protective power of *Belladonna*.

The mode he adopted of drawing the attention of physicians to his newly discovered prophylactic was singula. He announced for publication work on the subject, and advertised for subscribers promising to publish the work, which should reverse the name of the prophylactic, as soon as he got 300 subscribers, and in the mean time supplying to each subscriber a portion of the prophylactic, and demanding his opinion as to its efficacy. This unusual proceeding, which might be justified on the plea that Hahnemann wished to have the prophylactic tested more impartially than it would have been had he at once revealed the name of it, gave rise to a shower of bitter calumnies from his colleagues, who made little or no response to his offer, but loaded him with accusations of avarice and selfishness. Hahnemann revenged himself on his calcumniators, by publishing his pamphlet on scarlatina, wherein he revealed the name of the prophylactic, and the facts that led to his discovery. I need not remind you that the united testimony of almost all homoeopathic practitioners, and of the most distinguished of the allopaths, was favourable to the truth of Hahnemann's discovery. Indeed, nearly twenty years afterwards, whilst Hahnemann was residing in Leipzic, some physicians of that town complacently recommended the employment of *Belladonna* as a prophylactic for scarlet fever, as if they had just made the discovery, without alluding in the slightest way to the claims of the venerable sage in their midst, although they could scarcely fail to be known to them. But I am anticipating.

The hostility of the apothecaries and physician of Konigslutter drove him from that town in 1799. He purchased a large carriage or waggon, in which he packed all his property and family, and with a heavy heart bade adieu to Konigslutter, where fortune had at length begun to smile upon him, and where he had found leisure and opportunity to prosecute his interesting discoveries. Many of the inhabitants whose health he had been instrumental in, restoring or whose lives he had even saved by the discoveries of his genius during that fatal epidemic of scarlet fever, accompanied

him some distance on the road to Humburg, whither
he had resolved to proceed, and at length, with a blessing
for his services and a sigh for his hard lot, they bade
him God speed. And thus he journeyed on with all his
earthy possessions, and with all his family beside him.
But a dreadful accident befell the melancholy cortege.
Descending a precipitous part of the road, the waggon
was overturned, the driver thrown off his seat, his infant
son so injured that he died shortly afterwards and the
leg of one of his daughters fractured. He himself was
considerably bruised, and his property much demaged
by falling into a stream that ran at the bottom of the
road. With the assistance of some peasants they were
conveyed to the nearest village, where he was forced to
remain upwards of six weeks on his daughter's account,
at an expense that greatly lightened his not very well-
filled purse. At length he got in safety to Hamburg, but
finding little or nothing to do here, he removed to the
adjoining town of Altona. He did not, however, better
himself by the change, and not long after removed to
Mollen in Lauenburg; but the longing for his fatherland,
which he describes as being so strong in him, soon
drew him once more to Saxony. He planted himself in
Eulenburg, but the persecution of the superintend
physician of that place drove him thence after a short
sojourn. He wandered first to Machern, and thence to
Dessau, where we find him in 1803 publishing *a
monograph on the effects of coffee*, which he considered
as the source of many chronic diseases, and against
the use of which, as a common beverage, he inveighed
with much the same energy as our own first James did
against tobacco, previous to this, however, and during

his wanderings, he had translated several books from the English, and written various articles on his favourite idea of medical reform in Hufelands's Journal, denouncing ever more and more energetically the absurdities and errors of ordinary medical practise. One of the most remarkable articles in his style is his preface to a translation of a collection of medical prescriptions, published in 1800, which preface is the best antidote to the contents of the work itself. We can imagine his great soul fretting and fuming when the publisher, on whom he then almost entirely depended for subsistence, put into his hands the English original of this notable work, which contained ought but a collection of the abdominable and nonsensical compounds which he had been in weighing against for the last five years. We can fancy Hahnemann saying. *"Well, Sir, if you have more agreeable work to put me to hang this, I will do it; but mark, I stipulate to be allowed in write what preface I choose."* And such a preface it is the most marvellous preface surely that was; ever written for any book ! it is as though he had said, "Reader you have purchased this book thinking to find therein a royal road to the practice of physic, but you are miserably mistaken to believe there can be any such short cut; skill in practice can only be gained by careful, unwearied, and honest study; by having a perfect knowledge of the curative instruments you have to wield, and by an accurate observation of the characteristic symptoms of disease. As for the contents of this book, they are the grossest imposition ever palmed upon man, a confused jumble of unknown drugs—mostly poisons mixed together in what are called prescriptions, each ingredient of which is dignified by some imposing name that is meant to express the qualities it should possess and the part it should play, but none of which possesses the qualities attributed to it nor will obey, even in the slightest degree, the orders that are given it. Every prescription contains in it a multitude of anarchical elements that totally disqualify it for any orderly action whatever. The best counsel I can give you, my simple minded reader, is to put the main body of this book into the fire; but by all means preserve the preface; it may serve you as a standard for judging of the pretensions of similar pretentious books, of which there be, I am sorry to think, many, too many in the market just now, but which we shall do our best, with God's help, to rid the world of." I do not believe the publisher of this "**Arzneischatz**," or "**Treasury of Medicines**," would wish to give Hahnemann many more jobs of this kind to do, or if he did, he would doubtless resolve to bargain that no preface should be inserted. Indeed, we find that Hahnemann's translations came to rather an abrupt termination at this period, for, with the exception of a translation of the **Materia Medica** of the great **Albert von Haller**, which he executed in 1806, Hahnemann's works were hence forward all originals.

The years 1805 and 1806 were eventful ones for the development of the doctrine, and whilst he demolished the time honoured faith in the medicine of 3000 years, in his masterly little work entitled *A Esculapius in the Balance*, the temple of his own system, of which he had hitherto been only laying the foundations, commenced to exhibit some of those fair proportions which we now admire, by the appearance of the first sketch of a **Pure Materia Medica** which he gave to the world in Latin, and of that wonderful exposition of his whole doctrine, entitled **the Medicine of Experience**, which was published in 1806 in Hufeland's Journal.

And what was the reception this admirable work met with the most original, logical, and brilliant essay that had ever appeared on the art of medicine? A thousand captious objectors arose, who not being able to refute the masterly arguments brought forward by Hahnemann, fell to ridiculing the technicalities of the system; an easy task, since we all know that every new truth appears at first ridiculous. Nor was calumny silent. Hahnemann was loaded with most opprobious epithets because be introduced the custom, then unusual in Germany, of making the patients with whom he corresponded pay him for each epistolary consultation. This the facilities afforded by the arrangements of the German Post Office enabled him to do, and he was led to adopt it by the circumstance that so many sought his advice from mere curiosity or worse motives, without any thought or intention of paying, that he was driven to the adoption of what might be an unusual but was certainly not a reprehensible plan for securing the bonafides of his patients. A mistake he had made in his former chemical days was raked up from the limbo of forgotten things, and imputed to him as a gross crime, and a proof of his venality and dishonesty; though, in reality, the whole story redounds to his credit. During the period when he had temporarily abandoned medicine in disgust at its uncertainty, and had devoted himself solely to chemical and literary pursuits, he fancied he had discovered a new alkali, which he denominated pneum, and which he sold to those who wished to possess it. Subsequent investigation showed him that he had committed a mistake, and that the substance he had supposed to be a perfectly new matter was nothing but borax. He hastened to acknowledge his error, and lost no time in refunding to the purchasers the money he had received for it.

He was now settled in **Torgan**, and perceiving that his discoveries and labours met with nothing but opposition, contempt, and neglect from his medical brethren, disdaining to reply to any of the odious calumnies that were heaped upon him by those who should have been proud of him as their countryman and colleague, he discontinued writing in their medical journals, and appealed to the injustice of his professional brethren to the unprejudiced judgement of an enlightened public, and henceforth published his strictures on ancient medicine, and his projects for entitled the **Allgemeiner Anzeiger der Deutschen**. During the years 1808 and 1809, he published in that journal a succession of papers equal in terseness, vigour and originality to anything he had previously written, among which two deserve especial mention, viz., his essay on the value of the **Speculative System of Medicine**, and touching and earnest letter to Hufeland, whom he never ceased to love and esteem, though in every respect he was a much greater man and finer character than the Nester of German medicines, as Hufeland was called. The doctrines which were scornfully rejected by the **Scribes and Phairsees** of the old school found favour with public, and the number of his admirers and non-medical disciples increased from day to day. In 1810 he published the first edition of his immortal **Organon**, which was an amplification and extension of his **Medicine of Experience**, worked up with greater care, and put into a more methodical and aphoristic form, after the model of some of the Hippocratic writings.

With a wide-spread reputation he now re-entered Leipzic, where a crowd of patients and admirers flocked around him, and the flood-tide of fortune seemed at length to set in towards him. **Professor Hecker** of Berlin wrote, in 1810, a violent diatribe against the **Organon**, which displays more worth and untempered hostility than wit or good breeding, and was replied to in a vigorous manner by young **Frederick Hahnemann**, who undertook the defence of his father, for the latter treated all attacks, whether on his character or his works, with silent contempt; though it could not be said he viewed them with indifference, for their is every reason to believe the poisoned shafts of envy and calumny, rankled in his soul and communicated acerbity to a disposition that was naturally overflowing with love to his fellow-men. Hecker's attack was the sign for numerous others of the same nature, written with greater or less ability and with more or less fairness; but it would be wearisome to recapitulate even the titles of the articles and pamphlets that issued from the press intended by their authors to crush the presumptuous innovator.

However, this was not the effect they had. Hahnemann steadily pursued his course without condescending to notice the attacks of his adversaries, and in 1811 he published the first volume of the **Pure Materia Medica**, which contained the pathogenesis of the medicines he had been silently testing upon himself and friends, together with the symptoms he had called from various records of poisoning by the same substances. His earnest wish at this time was to found some college with hospital attached, for the purpose of indoctrinating the rising generation of physicians in homoeopathy, theoretically and practically; but this plan failing, he resolved to give a course of lectures upon the system to those medical men and students who wished to be instructed in it. In order to be allowed to do this, however, he had to pay a certain sum of money and defend a thesis before the Faculty of Medicine. To this regulation we are indebted for that able essay, **De Helleborismo veterum**, which no one can read without confessing that Hahnemann treats the subject in a masterly way and displays an amount of acquaintance with the writings of the Greek, Latin, Arabian and other physicians, from Hippocrates down his own time, that is possessed by few, and a power of philological criticism that has been rarely equalled. This thesis he defended on the 26th of June, 1812, and it drew from his adversaries an unwilling acknowledgment of his learning and genius, and from the impartial and worthy Dean of the Faculty a strong expression of admiration. When a candidate defends his thesis, he has what are called opponents among the examiners, who dispute the various opinions breached in the thesis; but the most of Hahnemann's opponents were schooled such an amiable state of mind by this display of learning, that they hastened to confess they were entirely of his way of thinking, while a few, who wished to say something for form's sake, merely expressed their dissent from some of Hahnemann's philological views. This trial, which his enemies had gain hoped would end in an exposure of the ignorance of the shallow charlation, trimphantly proved the superiority of Hahnemann over his opponents, even on their own territory, and was a brilliant inauguration of the lectures which he forthwith commenced to deliver to a circle of admiring students and grey headed old doctors, whom the fame of his doctrines and his learning attracted round him. He lectured twice a week, and from among the followers who gathered round him he selected a number to assist him in the labours of proving medicines, which he pursued without intermission. The vast amount of self-sacrifice, devotion, and endurance these labours must have required from him, those only who have attempted to prove medicines can form and idea of.

During his residence in Leipzic, from 1810 to 1821, he from time to time published valuable essays in the literary journal I have already alluded to, one of which was on a deadly form of typhus that broke out in 1814, in consequence of the disturbances caused by the stupendous military operations of that period, more particularly by the disorderly retreat of the French army from Russia. And he departed on one occasion from his usual habit, and wrote a couple of controversial articles upon the treatment of burns, for which he recommended warm applications in opposition to Professor Dzondi, who had advised the employment of cold water. A second edition of the Organon and five more volumes of Materia Medica appeared during this period, adding once to his fame and to the perfection of his system, which began to attract the attention of many physicians and immense numbers of the educated and upper classes.

The jealousy of his professional brethren, however, led them to incite the privileged guild of apothecaries to play the same game that had proved so successful in expelling Hahnemann from other places, and their machinations were only stayed for a time by the arrival in Leipzic of the celebrated **Austrian Field Marshal, Prince Schwarzenberg**, who came thither avowedly with the design of placing himself under Hahnemann's care, as his life was despaired of by the first practitioners of the old school. At first considerable amendment ensued, but his disease, which was some organic affection of the brain or heart, eventually had a fatal termination.

Of course a cry was now got up that Hahnemann's method hastened if it did not actually cause the death of illustrations commander, and the apothecaries, taking advantage of the unpopularity which this catastrophe, and the mode in which it was "improved" by his medical brethren, cast upon Hahnemann found now little difficulty in obtaining an injunction against his dispensing his own medicines. Hahnemann could not write prescriptions for his medicines, seeing that the privileged apothecaries did not keep them and could not be trusted with their preparation, as they were his bitterest foes. His practise was therefore gone, and though he was urgently advised to dispense his medicines secretly, yet he had too great a respect for the authority of the law to act contrary to the verdict of those whose business it was to enforce it, even although he believed that they misinterpreted its spirit. Nothing was left for him therefore but to quit Leipzic, a town which was now endured to him by many pleasing associations connected with the development of his great reform, and his fatherland, Saxony, now offered no place where the most illustrious of its sons could live in peace.

Under these discouraging circumstances the reigning prince of **Anhalt Coethen**, who was an ardent admirer of the system, offered Hahnemann an asylum in the tiny capital of his tiny dominions, and according to **Coethen Hahnemann** proceeded in 1821. It must have been with a heavy heart that he left Leipzic, the goal of his youth's ambition and the scene of his manhood's triumphs. It must have cost him a pang to leave that dear fatherland, for which he had always sighed in all his wanderings. To exchange the busy commercial and literary capital of northern Germany for the lifeless and dismal little town of a petty principality was but a sorry exchange indeed; and the deserted ill-paved streets and rude environs of the provincial town were a poor compensation for the lively and frequented promenades round Leipzic, where he used to walk every afternoon with his portly wife and numerous family. Though Leipzic has now the honour of containing his bronze effigies, and though Leipzic's magistrates and municipal authorities joined in the inauguration of Hahnemann's monument in 1851, this will hardly suffice to efface the strain of bigotry and intolerance that attaches to the town and its authorities by their expulsion of the greatest of Leipzic's citizen's in 1821.

The favour of the Duke, who appointed him Hofrath and physician in ordinary to his serene person and court, could scarcely make up to Hahnemann for the loss of the disciples whom he used to instruct and the friends who used to assist him in his provings; and his habits, which had never been very sociable, now become more than ever retired. After settling at Coethen he seldom crossed the threshold of his door except to visit his patron when he was sick; all the other patients who flocked to Coethen for his advice he saw at his own house, and his only walks were in a little garden at the back of his house, which he used jocularly to observe, though very narrow was infinitely high. Here he daily promenaded for a certain times as regularly as he had done in the pleasant Leipzic alleys, and every fine day he used to take a drive in his carriage into the country. He devoted himself entirely to practice and the development of his system. His amazing industry and perseverance never flagged an instant; he worked incessantly, it might be said. Here he published a **third**, a **fourth**, and a **fifth** edition of his **Organon** and a **second** and **third** edition of his **Materia Medica**, each time with great additions and careful revisions. Here also he wrote many articles for the literary journal before alluded to.

In 1827 he summoned to Coethen his two oldest and most esteemed disciples **Drs. Stapf** and **Gross**, and communicated to them his theory of the origin of chronic diseases and his discovery of a completely new series of medicaments for their cure, exhorting them to test the reality of his opinions and discoveries in their own practice. The next year the first and second volumes of his celebrated work on **Chronic diseases**, their peculiar nature and homoeopathic treatment, appeared. The doctrines therein inculcated were not received with implicit faith by all his disciples, for whilst some professed to perceive in them a discovery equal if not superior to that of the homoeopathic therapeutic law others were not satisfied that the deductions arrived at were justified by the facts on which they were professedly based. To Hahnemann's opponents his doctrine of chronic diseases was a fertile and inexhaustible theme for ridicule and obloquy, which he was usual paid no attention to, though his followers had now become so numerous that they began to take up the cudgels in their master's defence, and the medical press of Germany groaned with polemical articles respecting homoeopathy from both sides, of more or less ability. Since the year 1822 the homoeopathits had a quarterly journal, that contained many able and vigorous articles in support of Hahnemann's doctrines. A **third,** a **fourth**, and a **fifth** volume of **Chronic diseases**, containing extensive and valuable provings of new medicines, successively appeared during the following two years. The volume of these works can scarcely be over estimated, and they, with the **Materia Medica,** constitute the inexhaustible treasury on which the homoeopathic practitioner draws for the cure and relief of many diseases in which the allopathic appliances are important or hurtful.

On the 10th August, 1829, a large concourse of his disciples and admirers assembled at Coethen, for the purpose of celebrating the fiftieth anniversary of his reception of the Doctor's degree, and the dull little town was enlivened for a moment by the festivities of which it was the scene. The same day Hahnemann solemnly found the first **Homoeopathic Society**, under the name of the "**Central Society of German Homoeopathists**", which exists and flourishes to this day, and by whose exertions it was that the bronze statue was last year (1851) erected at Leipzic, as a grateful memento to its illustrious founder.

The success of homoeopathy, which now began to spread beyond the limits of Germany, and to make its way in other countries of Europe and in America, increased the bitterness and ferocity of the attacks of the partisans of the old school. They at length roused even the forbearance of Hahnemann, who published a pamphlet against his foes, entitled "**Allopathy : A Warning to all Sick Persons**," which, though undoubtedly in gross caricature of the system, turns into ridicule, has, like all good caricatures, an unmistakable though ludicrous likeness to the original in every feature, which must have rendered its sting all the more pungent.

The same year, 1831, the cholera invaded Germany from the East and on its approach, Hahnemann, guided by the unerring therapeutic rule he had discovered, at once fixed upon the remedies which should prove specifics for it, and caused directions to be printed, and distributed over the country by thousands so that on its actual invasion the homoeopathists and those who had received Hahnemann's directions were fully prepared for its treatment and prophylaxis, and thus there is no doubt many lives were saved, and many victims rescued from the pestilence. On all sides statements were published, testifying to the immense comparative success that had attended the employment of the means recommended by Hahnemann, before he had seen or treated a single case. This one fact speaks more for homoeopathy, and the truth of the law of nature on which the system is founded, than almost any other I could offer, viz., that Hahnemann, from merely reading a description of one of the most appealingly rapid and fatal diseases, could confidently and dogmatically say, such and such a medicine will do good in this stage of the disease; such and such other medicine in that; and that the united experience of hundreds of practitioners in all parts of Europe should bear practical testimony to the accuracy of Hahnemann's conclusions.

In 1830 Hahnemann lost his wife the mother of his numerous family, and the sharer of all the vicissitudes of his eventful life. It has been stated that his good lady had not the sweetest of tempers, and that she was somewhat of a Xantippe to our Socrates; but, as far as I can learn, there is no ground for this accusation. There is no doubt that she was a most affectionate wife and mother; but at the same time a strict disciplinarian, who asserted her supremacy over the domestic affairs and over her husband, in as far as he was part and parcel of the household; that Hahnemann loved and highly esteemed her we have ample evidence, from many passages in his letters, and from the testimony of his friends.

The death of his partner did not alter in any respect Hahnemann's **mode of life**; and his daughters, who had now attained the years of discretion, assumed the office of domestic supervision, vice **Mrs Hahnemann** deceased.

In 1835 **Mille Melanic d'Hervilly** came to Coethen, succeeded in captivating Hahnemann, then in his eightieth year, by the charms of her youth and beauty, and carried him off in triumph to Paris, where by her influence with **M. Gulzot** she obtained for him the authorization to practise. This second marriage, which took all his friends by surprise, is certainly a very unexpected denoucement in the last act of Hahnemann's life-drama. We trace with interest the progress of the man of science through his childhood's innocence, his youth's studious hours, his manhood's struggles with aversity, and indefatigable search after truth, until the final triumph and success of the aged philosopher. We note his habits of study, contemplation, and observation of nature; his retired, almost **unsocial life**; his devotion to the one great aim of his existence. We see him thus engaged up to a period of life exceeding the term of ordinary old age—when suddenly he takes a gay Parisian damsel to wife; the monotonous life of the dull country town and the accustomed seclusion of domestic retirement delight him no longer; and he hurries off to the capital of the *beau monde* with his youthful and elegant bride. This marriage, which comes upon us so abruptly, produced a total revolution in Hahnemann's habits and tastes. In Paris, we find him entertaining company and accepting invitations; frequenting the opera, and partaking moderately of the dissipations of the gay capital, and no longer confining his medical practise to the consultations at his own house, but visiting patients at their residences, like any other practitioner, which he had not done in Germany for more than twenty years previously. He seems to have entered on this novel course of life with great zest; and his new wife, to judge from his letters and the testimony of observers, rendered the latter years of his life extremely happy.

Notwithstanding this extreme change in his habits and occupations, he found time to make many and important additions to his great work on chronic diseases, of which he brought out a second edition after his removal to Paris, and it is said he was preparing for the press sundry other works of great importance to homoeopathy, which he was dissuaded from publishing by his wife. There is a tradition current among homoeo- pathists, that Mme. Hahnemann retains under lock and key, for her own private study doubtless, untold treasures of provings, cases, practical remarks, and new and revised editions of his works, which it would delight the hearts of all his disciples to see given to the world*.

---

* Thanks to Dr. Hachl's efforts that lost treasure has been secured. It consists of 54 case books containing the records of all patients treated by Hahnemann from 1799 to 1843; four large volumes of some 1500 pages each, alphabetically arranged repertories, none of which had ever been published; the sixth edition of Organon completely revised by Hahnemann till 1842 (since published in 1821 the English translation of this edition by W. Boericke, M.D.); some 1300 letters of physicians from all parts of the world, etc.........

Hahnemann survived his migration to Paris eight years and died there full of years and of honour, at the age of eightynine, on the 2nd July, 1843.

He was buried in the cemetery of **Montmartre**, and his body was attended to the grave by only four of his nearest relatives. We might have wished that man, who had acted such an important part in the world's history, had a less meagre attendance of his last resting place.

Such is a brief outline of the life and labours of Hahnemann, whose name, even by the admission of those most wildly opposed to his doctrines, must henceforth form an epoch in the history of medicine, as the founder of a school which has gained more adherents and roused up more assailants, written more books, and exercised a more important influence on the art of medicine, than any school or sect since the days of **Galen**.

The homoeopathic principle, as a law of therapeutics, is an immutable law of nature, and is altogether independent of any individual; but the homoeopathic system, or the doctrines and technicalities that have been agglomerated round that principle, bears the impress of the personality—the individuality of its author.

While, then, the principle bears the closet inspection, and gains ever more and more upon our belief and conviction the more searchingly we examine it, the system may naturally be expected to derive some of its characteristics from the peculiar mental constitution of the man who originated it; and hence it is that we find the homoeopathic school, as it is termed, while they bow unhesitatingly to the principle and to the logical deduction that flow from it, disputing with Hahnemann inch by inch the doctrines, and tenets, technicalities which he has had accumulated round this principle.

To facilitate our inquiries as to what parts of the system promulgated by Hahnemann belong to the domain of the unerring laws of nature, what derive a colouring and a bias from the individuality of the author, I think it is of great importance to endeavour to form a just estimate of his character and mental organization, and as I believe the circumstances of his life have exercised a considerable influence on his doctrines and precepts, and have contributed powerfully to the formation of his very remarkable character, I have not hesitated, at the risk of fatiguing you, to employ the time allotted for this first lecture in laying before you the sketch of his life just read, and I shall now, with your leave, turn to a consideration of the character and mental constitution of the man.

The most striking peculiarity of Hahnemann's mind was indomitable perseverance in following out the line of conduct he believed to be the true one, notwith-standing every difficulty and discouragement. Thus we have seen him as a boy persisting in devoting himself to study in spite of the opposition of his father and poring over his books by the light of his **contraband oil**, in the primitive lamp of his own construction. In later years we find him eking out the means of his support whilst studying medicine, by teaching others his surreptitiously acquired knowledge, and translating books from various languages, with contents of many of which he could have had little or no sympathy. It is related of him that he sat up every alternate night, and, in order to enable himself to do so, acquired that inveterate habit of smoking, tobacco, which be continued to indulge in to the last. The means he took to chase away his slumbers in his youth thus became in after years the only luxury in which he indulged.

This perseverance was conspicuous in the means he adopted of pursuing his studies in the great **medical school of Vienna**, for which he carefully accumulated as much money as was sufficient to maintain him in that expensive capital for some time, he had not been defrauded of it, and thereby obliged to cut his studies prematurely short, and accept of a post in the remote town of **Hermannstadt**. As further proofs of this iron perseverance, I have only to remind you of his undeviating efforts to follow up the truth he discovered, and to perfect the system he originated, undeterred for one instant by the hard necessities of poverty, or by the sneers and persecutions of those who should most have befriended and encouraged him, his professional brethren. The inveterate and incensing persecution to which he was subjected from the very commencement of his career and which increased in intensity as he developed his peculiar and novel doctrines, had not the slightest effect in making him relax in the least degree from his endeavours. His very first work of any importance, that on Syphilis, was, as he himself tells us, the subject of the most outrageous vituperations and any abuse. Though this work was published long before he had any idea of homoeopathy, the views he promulgated with reference to the destruction by caustics of the primary sore, and the employment of very small quantities of a new mercurial preparation, running counter as they did to the prevalent notions on the subject, called forth the most unwarrantable abuse from his critics. The same thing happened on the publication of his Essay on a new Principle; and every other step in the progress of his great and beneficent discovery was greeted with similar discouragement. In 1799, the more practical annoyance of the apothecaries persecution was called into play, and the intrigues of his enemies drove him from place to place. With a large and increasing family to provide for, this system of persecution must have been the most painful and annoying to his feelings that could be devised. Wherever he went the espionage of the **German Worshipful Company of Apothecaries** accompanied him, and the moment he was detected dispensing his own medicines, a complaint was made on the part of that privileged guild that he was interfering with their vested rights. And it was no difficult matter to get evidence against him, for he held it to be indispensable to the right practice of his art to have the command over his own tools, and scorned to conceal that he dispensed his own medicines. Although all this persecution did not tend to him swerve one jot from the line of conduct he had marked out for himself, it no doubt contributed greatly to his adoption of those secluded and recluse habits he was noted for in afterlife, to render him intolerant of contradiction, and to make him view with suspicion, if not with envy, any one who ventured to differ from him by ever so little. Many of the acts which this disposition led him to commit are greatly to be lamented. Thus be took upon himself to summon to Coethen the Homoeopathic Society he had founded only three years previously, though the place of meeting had been fixed for Leipzic, because he was told that some of his doctrines were opposed by some of its members; and the next year he pronounced the dissolution of the Society on the same grounds. His intolerance for those who differed from him latterly attained to such a height, that he used to say, **"He who does not walk on exactly the same line with me, who diverges, if it be but the breath of straw, to the right or to the left, is an apostate and a traitor, and with him I will have nothing to do**." **Dr. Gross**, who was one of his most industrious disciples and enjoyed his most perfect intimacy, having lost a child, wrote in the sorrow of a bereaved parent to Hahnemann, and said that his loss had taught him that homoeopathy did not suffice in every case; this gave great offence to Hahnemann, **who never forgave Gross for this remark, and never afterwards restored him to his favour**. The hospital that had been established in Leipzic by private subscription was also the scene of Hahnemann's intolerant spirit, for he never rested satisfied until the talented and zealous physician, **Dr. M. Muller**, who had the charge of it, and who performed the duties most efficiently and without payment, but who did not please Hahnemann because he ventured to exercise an independent judgement, was replaced by one entirely disposed to swear in **verba magistri**, with a salary of

300 thalers per anum. This spirit of intolerance of any difference of opinion on the part of those professing to be his disciples, which showed itself in many different ways, was doubtless partly occasioned by the violent opposition and persecution he had met with, and which had led him to retire as it were within himself, and adopt that almost hermit-life which we have seen him leading, whereby his own ideas not being modified or enlarged by the collision of independent minds with his own, always bore the distinctive characteristics of his own peculiar mental organization sharply defined, and anything that did not chime in exactly with his own standard for the time being was looked upon by him with suspicion and dislike. The reports, insinuations, and misrepresentations of those few persons who retained his intimacy by agreeing with him in everything he said, had also, it would seem, the effect of making his judgements on others more harsh than they would have been had he known them or suffered them to discuss with him their ideas. It should also be mentioned, his confidence in others had on several occasions received rude shocks, more especially in the case of a young physician of the name of **Robbi**, who insinuated himself into his intimacy by feighned respect and admiration for his genius, and subsequently turned round and was one of the foremost in ridiculing the system of the man for whom he had expressed such esteem. This circumstance, which occurred soon after his arrival in Leipzic, no doubt made him suspicious and impatient of the opposition of others. I am of opinion that it would have greatly contributed to the more general adoption of homoeopathy had Hahnemann been

more a man of the world, and had he taken into his
confidence some of those of his followers who were
distinguished for their independence of thought and
proficiency in the medical sciences. Homoeopathy would
in that case not have presented such a harsh contrast,
and stood in such violent antagonism to the old system
of medicine; for what was good and true in the latter
would have been adopted and amalgamated with the
reformed system to its advantage; and the improve-
ments, and discoveries in physiology, pathology, and
chemistry would have probably been made use of by
Hahnemann for the development of his system, had
these not proceeded from members of a party that had
declared war to the knife against Hahnemann and the
new school, ruptured every bond of amity between them.
Who can doubt that the inveterate enmity and persecution of the apothecaries had its certain amount of
influence in giving a bias to Hahnemann's mind on the
subject of the dose, and that it ultimately led to that
Procrustean standard for regulating the dose which
Hahnemann adopted, without sufficient grounds as I
believe? Who can doubt that the forced retirement of
Hahnemann, and the unfortunate resolution he adopted
of never visiting patients, must have latterly confined
his practice almost entirely to one class of patients,
those affected with chronic diseases, and that had he
seen more acute diseases, his practice would have been
considerably modified? The persecution of the
apothecaries began in 1799. Previous to this time
Hahnemann had given material and palpable doses, as
we learn from the cases he published anterior to that
date. In 1800 we first meet with anything like

infinitesimals, and these only in certain cases. As the opposition of the apothecaries become more violent, and the injury they inflicted on him, pecuniarily and otherwise, more severe, Hahnemann's doses became more and more refined and attenuated, until at length we find him stating that the mere smelling at a globule is not only sufficient but the best of all methods of administering the remedy; and he adds, with marked emphasis, that this will enable us to dispense entirely with the apothecary's services. When he got out of the sphere of the apothecaries' influence and annoyance he entirely altered his mode of giving the remedy and the method he adopted in Paris, which I have elsewhere described, is a much nearer approximation to the method of the dominant school.

But although the persecution of Hahnemann is to be regretted for the unfortunate influence it exercised on his doctrines in some respects, yet it is probably that on the whole this persecution was altogether disadvantageous to the internal development of the new system. The myth of Prumetheus chained to the solitary rock with the vulture growing at his liver is an emblem of the fate that awaits all who have the presumption to steal celestial fire; they are mostly condemned to solitude, their great minds can find no companionship among the common herd of mankind, and they are incessantly preyed upon by the ever-greedy vulture of envious detraction. Perhaps it is best for the new truths that their discoverers should be so treated. Their isolation and forced retirement from the world enable them to work more constantly at their subject and to developed it by the light of their own great minds, unswayed by the well-meaning but shallow friends, who are generally the most officious and persevering in their injudicious suggestions. Though, by the enforced intellectual solitude on the part of the discoverers of new truths, the systems they build-up may appear to be deficient in catholicity, and to bear too prominently the stamp of their authors' individuality, yet, on the other hands, there is no fear of their truths being lost aimed a medley of distracting doubts and irrelevant fancies, that would not fail to suggest themselves to the various minds of multitude of learned pundits. The persecutions endured by the pioneers of truth serve only to stimulate them more so to work out and perfect their truth, that their very enemies and persecutors shall be forced ultimately to bow down before it. While the sham melts away like snow before the fire of persecution, the truth is only rendered more bright and more compact by it, as the soft iron only becomes steel by passing through the furnace. That Hahnemann felt and felt deeply the unjust calcumnies and unceasing persecution to which he was subjected we have ample evidence from various passages in his works from the year 1800 onwards. Among the papers found at his death one bore the following inscription, intended as an epitaph on his tomb, which reads live the last sigh of a martyr—liber tendem quiesco.

Another quality of Hahnemann's mind conscientiousness, is strikingly displayed in his abandoning the lucrative practise of medicine when his faith was shaken in it and supporting his family for some time upon the proceeds of his chemical discoveries, and by the tenfold greater labour of translating books for the publisher. This quality is also shown in his refusal to adopt any mode of avoiding the persecutions of the apothecaries, which he might readily have done, either by setting up an apothecary of his own or by dispensing his medicines secretly. Another, if possible still more striking trait of conscientiousness which I have not found alluded to elsewhere, is this. After his first discovery of the homoeopathic therapeutic law, he contented himself for some years with making a collection of the morbid effects of various poisonous and medicinal substance from the writings and observations of the more ancient and the modern toxicologists and experimenters. In this way he collected together à tolerable pathogenesis of many powerful substances, and on this basis he endeavoured to practise. He published the results of his first trials of his system upon these data in 1796 and the two following years. But he soon found that the records of the toxicologists and others were inadequate to afford him sufficiently accurate pictures of morbid states corresponding to the natural diseases he had to treat, and he saw that there was nothing for it but to test the medicines and poisons accurately, carefully, and systematically upon the healthy individual. As yet he knew not if such trails might not be fraught with danger to his constitution and shorten life; but he did not shrink from what he considered a sacred duty, and he boldly set about the gigantic task—a task, I may safely say, from which any ordinary mind would have recoiled in dismay. How he executed his task I need not relate. The ten volumes of provings he has left us are an eternal

monument to his energy, perseverance, conscientiousness, and self-sacrifice. "When," say he, "**we have to
do with an art whose end is the saving of human
life, any neglect to make ourselves thoroughly
masters of it becomes a crime** !"

We may form some idea of Hahnemann's immense
industry when we consider that he proved about ninety
different medicines, that he wrote upwards of seventy
original works on chemistry and medicine, some of which
were in several thick volumes, and translated about
twenty-four works from the English, French, Italian,
and Latin, on chemistry medicine, agriculture, and
general literature, many of which were in more than
one volume. Besides this he attended to the duties of
an immense practice, corresponding and consulting, and
those who know the care and time he expanded on
every case, the accuracy with which he registered every
symptom, and the carefulness with which he sought
for the proper remedy, will be able to estimate what a
Herculean labour a large practice so conducted must
have been. When I add that he was an accomplished
classical scholar and philologist, and that he had more
than a superficial acquaintance with botany, astronomy,
meteorology, and geography, we shall be forced to
acknowledge that his industry and working powers
bordered on the marvellous.

His goodness of heart and generosity appear on
various occasions. In the fragment of autobiography I
have before alluded to, after relating that he was
swindled out of the hard earned gains by means of
which he hoped to pursue his medical studies in Vienna,

he says that the person who injured him was afterwards sorry for what he had done, so he freely forgives him, and will not mention either his name or the circumstances of the transaction. His enemies and some of his professed friends have accused him of avarice, founding this charge on the fact that he demanded high fees, made his corresponding patients pay for the consultation on receipt of the letter, and that he lived in a style not suited to his wealth. His frequent struggles with the direst poverty had no doubt taught him, by many cruel lessons, the value of money, and we can scarcely wonder that he was rather economical and saving, more especially as he had a large family, nine of whom were daughters, from whom he might any day be cut off and whom he would not like to leave portionless. That this was his real motive is evident from the circumstance that when he left Coethen for Paris he divided his fortune, amounting to 60,000 thalers, or about £ 10,000 sterling, among his family. If he took large fees he did so both because he had a very high idea of the dignity of his profession, and because he well knew the value of the services he rendered to his patients, and the amount of labour he had undergone in order to be enabled to render such services. To the poor he was liberal, in giving them the benefit of his advice gratuitously. As for the other charge brought against him of making the patients pay for the consultation on receipt of the letter, I think that was an arrangement which concerned Hahnemann's patients alone, and if they did not object to it, surely his colleagues had no occasion to find fault. Hahnemann, rather deserved the thanks than the censure of his colleagues for devising and introducing a method whereby the just interests of the profession were protected.

As to his religious principles, Hahnemann was brought up in the Lutheran persuasion, but he could not be said to have adopted the tenets of that or any other sect of Christians. His principles, as we gather them from his works were nearly these : **He believed in the ruling providence of an all good and all bountiful and God, and he held that every man was bound to his utmost to benefit each was endowed.** He traced every good thing to the hand of the almighty and beneficent God, to whom he always gave all the glory for all the good he was enabled to confer on his brethren of mankind, and denied to himself any merit for what he had done.

"One word more," he say writing to stapf in 1816, "be as sparing as possible with your praises. I do not like them. I feel that I am only an honest, straightforward man, who does no more than his duty".

Again, in his famous letter to Hufeland, he writes; "If experience should show you that my method is the best, then make use of it for the benefit of humanity and give God the glory!"

Here is a striking sentence indicative of his sense of the high dignity of our profession. He is alluding to his discovery of the pro-phylatic for scarlet fever : "The furtherance of every means, be it ever so small, that can save human life, that can bring health and security, (a God of love invented this blessed and most wondrous of arts) should be a sacred object to the true physician;

chance or the labour of a physician has discovered this one. Away, then, with all grovelling passions at the altar of this sublime Godhead, whose priests we are!"

Here his emotion respecting the character of the offices of doctor and sick-nurse in the time of plague and pestilence. They are, he writes, "two persons ordained by God, and placed, like Uriah in the battle, in the thickest of the light—forlorn hopes quite close to the advancing enemy, without any hours of relief from their irksome guard—two very much misunderstood beings, who sacrifice themselves at hard earned wages for the public weal, and, in order to obtain a civic crown, brave the life-destroying, poisoned atmosphere, deafened by the cries of agony and the groans of death."

There is not a work of Hahnemann's which is not pervaded by the spirit of reverence for the Dietary, whose humble instrument he feels himself to be, and love for his fellow-creatures, with which his truly benevolent heart overflows : "Oh, that it were mine!" he exclaims, after an examination of all the futile systems that had been proposed and adopted for the cure of diseases— "Oh, that it were mine to direct the better portion of the medical world, who can fell for the sufferings of our brethren of mankind and long to know how to relieve them, to those purer principles which lead directly to the desired goal ! Infamy be the award of history to him who, by deceit and fiction, maims this art of ours, which is intended to succour the wretched ! All compensating, divine self-approval, and an unfading civic crown to him who helps to make our art more beneficial to mankind!"

This he said in 1808, when the great truth was gradually developing itself under his hands. After thirty years spent in laboriously working out his system, and practically demonstrating that his were indeed those purer principles whereby the cure of diseases was most easily and safely effected, he was able to make this solemn declaration.

"My conscience is clear : it bears me witness that I have ever sought the welfare of suffering humanity, that I have always done and taught what seemed to me best, and that I have never had recourse to any allo-pathic procedures to comply with the wishes of my patients, and to prevent them leaving me. I love my fellow creatures and the repose of my conscience too much to act in that manner. Those who follow my example will be able, as I am, on the verge of the grave, to wait with tranquillity and confidence till the time comes when they must lay down their soul to a God whose omnipotence must strike terror into the heart of the wicked !"

The abnegation of all merit to himself for his many and irksome labours to perfect his art, and the humble acknowledgment of his gratitude and reliance on God, are strikingly shown in his memorable words upon his death-bed, the last utterance of his of which we have any record. Whilst suffering much from the pain and difficulty of breathing that attended his last fatal illness, his wife said to him. "As you in your laborious life have alleviated the sufferings of so many, and have yourself endured so much, surely Providence owes you a remission of all your sufferings." To which the dying sage replied, "My ! and why me? Man here below works according to the gifts and strength Providence has given him, and it is only before the fallible tribunal of man that degrees of merit are acknowledged, not so before that of God; God owes me nothing, but I owe Him much—yes everything."

Of all historical characters Hahnemann most nearly resembles the great religious reformer of the sixteenth century, Luther, to whom he was fond of comparing himself. We find in both the same energy and perseverance, the same dauntless proclamation of the truth, however disagreeable to constituted authorities, the same unflinching courage under the most annoying and wearing-out persecutions, the same cutting sarcasm and power of caricature when stung into retaliation by the machinations of their enemies, and the same constant trust in Providence and assurance of the ultimate triumph of their principles. I cannot forbear quoting a passage from a letter of Hahnemann's that shows at once his independence of all extraneous aid for the spread of his doctrines, and his confidence of their eventual general adoption.

"Our art," says he, "needs no political leave, no worldly badges of honour, in order to become something. Amid all the rank and unsightly weeds that flourish round about it, it grows gradually from a small acorn to a slender tree; already its lofty sumit overtops the rank vegetation around it. Only have patience ! It strikes its roots deep underground, gains strength imperceptibly, but all the more certainly, and in due time it will grow up to a lofty God's oak, stretching its great arms, that no longer bend to the storm far away into all religions of the earth, and mankind, who have hitherto been tormented, will be refreshed under its beneficent shadow !"

In its effects upon the established school of traditional medicine, the reformation of Hahnemann strongly resembles that of Luther on the **Roman Catholic Church**. Abused, vilified, persecuted, the young medical school has gone on gathering strength and securing the support of men distinguished for their learning and rank, until at length it has become a formidable rival to the antiquated system, which it threatens every day to extinguish. As Luther's reformation sapped the foundations of the Roman hierarchy, so Hahnemann's has more than shaken the stability of the temple of Hippocrates, which it will eventually overthrow completely, and more effectually than Luther did the ancient Church, for experimental science is more sweeping in its effects than theological, and never rests until the last pillar of error is overthrown. As the Reformation had its pretenders and its fanatics, so has Homoeopathy its charlatans and its bigots; but as the impartial historian will not confound the errors and delusions of the erratic religionists will the Reformation, so may we hope that the extravagant fancies and theories that have arisen out of Homoeopathy may not be confounded with the real spirit of Hahnemann's great medical reform. Almost every great truth has its unworthily adherents, who like the parasitical plant, stifle and disfigure that whereto they cling and whereby alone they exist but as the great oak survives and remains erect the monarch of the forest, long after generations of those inferior creatures to which it gave support have withered away and crumbled into dust, so the truth that Hahnemann revealed will outlive the memory of its unworthy parasites, and emerge from their unwholesome embrace a stately tree, a beacon of hope and a source of health and happiness to hundreds of unborn generations of suffering mankind.

Whilst pointing out the peculiarities in life and character of Hahnemann which we may presume to have exercised an influence upon his doctrines practice, I think the sketch I have given will suffice to show, from the whole course Hahnemann's life, from the magnanimity and fortitude with which he endured poverty in order to pursue the one great aim of his existence, from the sacrifices he made for the cause of truth, and from the devotion with which he subjected himself for a long series of years to the most unpleasant and hazardous experiments, for the purpose of perfecting his system, that its author was formed to the stuff that the world's worthies are made of and that if heroic constancy, amid the most discouraging circumstances, to one grand aim—that of benefiting humanity—constitutes a hero, Hahnemann eminently deserves to rank with the greatest of them, and the system originated by such a man merits the attention and study of all who are occupied with the cure of disease.

When the passions and prejudices engendered in the atmosphere of controversy shall have subsided, can we, who know the excellence of his system, doubt that the judgement of an impartial posterity will reverse the

condemnation of the packed jury of prejudiced contem-
poraries, and award a niche in the temple of fame, among
the greatest of the world's heroes and benefactors, to
the father of Rational Physic Samuel Hahnemann ?*

————◆————

* Introductory lecture delivered by Dr. Dudgeon at Hahnemann
Hospital, London during the sessions 1852-53.

FREE CATALOGUE COUPON

Yes, I am interested in Health Harmony titles. Please rush me the catalogue.

FREE CATALOGUE ORDER FORM
(Write in Capitals)

Name ....

Complete Mailing Address ....

....

....

....

....

.... Pin....................................

Ph. (Res.) .... Ph. (Off.) ....

E-mail. ....

Date ....   Signature

Mail this coupan to

HEALTH 🌳 HARMONY
an Imprint of

B. JAIN PUBLISHERS (P) LTD.
1921, Chuna Mandi, St. 10th Paharganj, New Delhi-110 055
Ph.: 3670572, 3670430, 3683200, 3683300
Fax: 011-3610471 & 3683400
Website: www.bjainbooks. com, Email:bjain@vsnl.com

SUBSCRIPTION COUPON

Yes, I want to subscribe to The Homoeopathic Heritage.

SUBSCRIPTION RATES FOR ONE YEAR

OVERSEAS CUSTOMERS

BANGLADESH	PAKISTAN	REST OF THE WORLD
$ 18/-	$ 32/-	$ 40/-

INDIAN CUSTOMERS

INDIA	NEPAL	BHUTAN
Rs. 200/-	Rs. 200/-	Rs. 200/-

MODE OF PAYMENT

For India, Nepal & Bhutan by M.O., Bank Draft or Cheque payable at Delhi, New Delhi in favour of **B. Jain Publishers (P) Ltd.,** 1921/10, Chuna Mandi, Paharganj, Post Box 5775, New Delhi-55, India.

For Overseas by International Money Order or Bank Draft in favour of **B. Jain Publishers Overseas,** 1920, Street No. 10th, Chuna Mandi, Post Box 5775, Paharganj, New Delhi - 110 055, India.

SUBSCRIPTION ORDER FORM
(Write in Capitals)

Name ....

Complete Mailing Address ....

....

....

.... Pin ....

Ph. (Res.) .... Ph. (Off.) ....

E-mail ....

I am remitting Rs./US$ .... by M.O./Bank Draft/Cheque

Date ....   Signature